NURSING DIAGNOSIS HANDBOOK

BETTY J. ACKLEY

citalopram

sye-tal-o-pram

Apo-Citalopram

CeleXA

Grouping

PHARMACOTHERAPEUTIC: Serotonin reuptake inhibitor.

CLINICAL: Antidepressant.

■ BLACK BOX ALERT ■ Increased danger of self-destructive reasoning and conduct

in youngsters, teenagers, youthful grown-ups 18–24 yrs with significant burdensome jumble, other mental problems.

Try not to mistake CeleXA for CeleBREX, Cerebyx, Ranexa, or ZyPREXA.

Employments

Treatment of gloom. OFF-LABEL: Treatment of liquor misuse, diabetic

neuropathy, over the top impulsive problem, smoking discontinuance, GAD, alarm

jumble.

Safeguards

Contraindications: Hypersensitivity to citalopram, utilization of MAOIs expected to

treat mental problems (simultaneously or inside 14 days of ceasing by the same token citalopram or MAOI), commencement in pts getting linezolid or methylene blue.

Simultaneous use with pimozide. Alerts: Elderly, hepatic/renal impedance,

seizure issue. Not suggested in pts with inherent long QT disorder,

bradycardia, ongoing MI, uncompensated HF, hypokalemia, or hypomagnesemia;

pts at high danger of self destruction.

Activity

Squares take-up of the synapse serotonin at CNS presynaptic neuronal

films, expanding its accessibility at postsynaptic receptor destinations.

Remedial Effect: Relieves indications of sorrow.

Pharmacokinetics

Very much consumed after PO organization. Protein restricting: 80%. Widely

utilized in liver. Discharged in pee. Half-life: 35 hrs.

Life expectancy contemplations

Pregnancy/Lactation: Distributed in bosom milk. Youngsters: May cause

expanded anticholinergic impacts, hyperexcitability. Old: More touchy to

anticholinergic impacts (e.g., dry mouth), bound to encounter unsteadiness, sedation, disarray, hypotension, hyperexcitability.

Associations

Medication: CYP2C19 inhibitors (e.g., fluconazole), different meds

dragging out QT span (e.g., amiodarone, azithromycin, ciprofloxacin,

haloperidol) may expand hazard of QT prolongation. Linezolid, MAOIs (e.g.,

phenelzine, selegiline), triptans may cause serotonin disorder (fervor,

diaphoresis, unbending nature, hyperthermia, autonomic hyperactivity, trance like state).

Natural: Gotu kola, kava, SAMe, St. John's wort, valerian may increment CNS despondency. St. John's wort might expand hazard of serotonin

disorder. FOOD: None known. LAB VALUES: May diminish serum sodium.

Accessibility (Rx)

Oral Solution: 10 mg/5 mL. Tablets: 10 mg, 20 mg, 40 mg.

Organization/dealing with

PO

• Give regardless of food.

Signs/courses/dose

Note: Doses more noteworthy than 40 mg not suggested.

Sadness

PO: ADULTS (under 60 yrs old enough): Initially, 20 mg once every day in the

morning or evening. May increment in 20-mg increases at timespans less

than 1 wk. Most extreme: 40 mg/day. Old (60 yrs old enough or more established): 20 mg

when every day. Greatest: 20 mg/day.

Portion Modification

Hepatic hindrance; helpless metabolizers of CYP2C19; corresponding utilization of

CYP2C19 inhibitors: 20 mg once day by day. Greatest: 20 mg/day.

Measurements in Renal Impairment

Gentle to direct impedance: No portion change. Serious hindrance: Use

alert.

Incidental effects

Continuous (21%–11%): Nausea, dry mouth, sleepiness, a sleeping disorder, diaphoresis.

Infrequent (8%–4%): Tremor, looseness of the bowels, unusual discharge, dyspepsia,

exhaustion, tension, heaving, anorexia. Uncommon (3%–2%): Sinusitis, sexual

brokenness, feminine issue, stomach torment, unsettling, diminished moxie.

Unfriendly impacts/harmful responses

Excess showed as wooziness, laziness, tachycardia, disarray, seizures,

torsades de pointes, ventricular tachycardia, unexpected demise. Serotonin condition

or on the other hand neuroleptic harmful condition (NMS)– like responses have been accounted for.

Nursing contemplations

Benchmark appraisal

Hepatic/renal capacity tests, blood counts ought to be performed intermittently for

pts on long haul treatment. Notice, record conduct. Evaluate mental status,

thought content, rest design, appearance, interest in climate. Screen for bipolar confusion.

Intercession/assessment

Direct self-destructive danger pt intently during early treatment (as gloom decreases,

energy level improves, expanding self destruction potential). Evaluate appearance,

conduct, discourse design, level of interest, mind-set.

Patient/family educating

- Do not quit taking prescription or increment dose.

- Avoid liquor.

- Avoid undertakings that require readiness, engine abilities until reaction to sedate is set up.

• Report demolishing wretchedness, self-destructive ideation, strange changes in conduct.

clarithromycin

kla-rith-roe-mye-sin

Apo-Clarithromycin

Biaxin

Biaxin XL

PMS-Clarithromycin

Order

PHARMACOTHERAPEUTIC: Macrolide.

CLINICAL: Antibiotic.

Try not to mistake clarithromycin for Claritin, clindamycin, or

erythromycin.

Employments

Treatment of helpless diseases because of C. pneumoniae, H. influenzae, H.

parainfluenzae, H. pylori, M. catarrhalis, M. avium, M. pneumoniae, S. aureus,

S. pneumoniae, S. pyogenes, including bacterial worsening of bronchitis, otitis

media, intense maxillary sinusitis, Mycobacterium avium complex (MAC), pharyngitis, tonsillitis, H. pylori duodenal ulcer, local area procured

pneumonia, skin and delicate tissue contaminations. Anticipation of MAC illness. OFFLABEL: Prophylaxis of infective endocarditis, pertussis, Lyme sickness.

Safety measures

Contraindications: Hypersensitivity to clarithromycin, other macrolide

anti-microbials. History of QT prolongation or ventricular arrhythmias, including

torsades de pointes. History of cholestatic jaundice or hepatic debilitation with

earlier utilization of clarithromycin. Attendant use with colchicine (in pts with renal/hepatic hindrance), lovastatin, simvastatin, pimozide, ergotamine,

dihydroergotamine. Alerts: Hepatic/renal hindrance, older with serious

renal hindrance, myasthenia gravis, coronary course sickness. Pts in danger of

delayed heart repolarization. Stay away from use with uncorrected electrolytes (e.g.,

hypokalemia, hypomagnesemia), clinically huge bradycardia, class IA or

III antiarrhythmics (see Classification).

Activity

Ties to ribosomal receptor destinations of defenseless organic entities, hindering protein combination of bacterial cell divider. Restorative Effect: Bacteriostatic; might be

bactericidal with high measurements or truly vulnerable microorganisms.

Pharmacokinetics

All around retained from GI plot. Protein restricting: 65%–75%. Broadly disseminated

(but CNS). Used in liver. Basically discharged in pee. Not eliminated by

hemodialysis. Half-life: 3–7 hrs; metabolite, 5–9 hrs (expanded in renal

debilitation).

Life expectancy contemplations

Pregnancy/Lactation: Unknown whenever circulated in bosom milk. Kids: Safety

also, adequacy not set up in pts more youthful than 6 mos. Older: Age-related

renal debilitation might require measurement change.

Communications

Medication: May expand fixations, harmfulness of carBAMazepine, colchicine,

digoxin, ergotamine, theophylline, sildenafil, tadalafil, vardenafil.

Atorvastatin, efavirenz, rifabutin, rifAMPin might diminish plasma

fixation. May build impact of warfarin. May diminish centralization of zidovudine. Atazanavir, ritonavir might build grouping of

clarithromycin. Home grown: St. John's wort might diminish plasma fixation.

FOOD: None known. LAB VALUES: May build serum BUN, ALT, AST,

antacid phosphatase, LDH, creatinine, PT. May diminish WBC.

Accessibility (Rx)

Oral Suspension (Biaxin): 125 mg/5 mL, 250 mg/5 mL. Tablets (Biaxin): 250

mg, 500 mg.

Tablets (Extended-Release [Biaxin XL]): 500 mg.

Organization/dealing with

PO

- Give quick delivery tablets, oral suspension regardless of food.

- Give q12h (as opposed to twice every day).

- Shake suspension a long time before each utilization.

- Extended-discharge tablets ought to be given with food.

- Do not break, smash, disintegrate, or partition broadened discharge tablets.

Signs/courses/dose

Regular Dosage Range

PO: ADULTS, ELDERLY: 250–500 mg q12h or 1,000 mg once every day (expanded delivery tablets). Kids 6 MOS AND OLDER: (ImmediateRelease): 7.5 mg/kg q12h. Most extreme: 500 mg/portion.

Dose in Renal Impairment

CrCl under 30 mL/min: Reduce portion by half and manage more than once

every day. HD: Administer portion after dialysis complete.

Mix with atazanavir or ritonavir

CrCl 30–60 mL/min Decrease portion by half

CrCl under 30 mL/min Decrease portion by 75%

Dose in Hepatic Impairment

No portion change.

Incidental effects

Intermittent (6%–3%): Diarrhea, sickness, adjusted taste, stomach torment. Uncommon

(2%–1%): Headache, dyspepsia.

Unfavorable impacts/harmful responses

Anti-infection related colitis, different superinfections (stomach cramps, serious

watery loose bowels, fever) may result from adjusted bacterial equilibrium in GI parcel.

Hepatotoxicity, thrombocytopenia happen seldom.

Nursing contemplations

Standard evaluation

Question pt for hypersensitivities to clarithromycin, erythromycins.

Mediation/assessment

Screen every day example of gut action, stool consistency. Gentle GI impacts may

be average, yet expanding seriousness might show beginning of anti-infection related

colitis. Be ready for superinfection: fever, heaving, loose bowels, butt-centric/genital

pruritus, oral mucosal changes (ulceration, torment, erythema).

Patient/family instructing

- Continue treatment for full length of treatment.

• Doses ought to be uniformly dispersed.

• Biaxin might be taken regardless of food. Take Biaxin XL with food.

• Report serious loose bowels.

clevidipine

clev-eye-di-peen

Cleviprex

Grouping

PHARMACOTHERAPEUTIC: Dihydropyridine calcium channel blocker.

CLINICAL: Antihypertensive.

Try not to mistake clevidipine for amlodipine, cladribine, clofarabine,

clozapine, or Cleviprex with Claravis.

Employments

The executives of hypertension when oral treatment isn't doable or not alluring.

Safeguards

Contraindications: Hypersensitivity to clevidipine. Sensitivity to soy or egg

items; strange lipid digestion (e.g., intense pancreatitis, lipoid nephrosis,

pathologic hyperlipidemia whenever joined by hyperlipidemia), serious aortic stenosis. Alerts: HF; pt with problems of lipid digestion.

Activity

Causes intense blood vessel vasodilation by hindering the flood of calcium during

depolarization in blood vessel smooth muscle. Helpful Effect: Decreases mean

blood vessel pressure (MAP) by lessening fundamental vascular opposition.

Pharmacokinetics

Generally and quickly appropriated. Full recuperation of helpful B/P happens 5–15

min. after suspension. Beginning of impacts: 2–4 min. Processed through hydrolysis by esterases in blood and extravascular tissue. Protein restricting: 99.5%. Discharged

in pee (74%), excrement (22%). Half-life: 15 min.

Life expectancy contemplations

Pregnancy/Lactation: Unknown whenever disseminated in bosom milk. May push down

uterine withdrawals during work and conveyance. Youngsters: Safety and adequacy not

set up in pts more youthful than 18. Old: Start at low finish of dosing range.

May encounter more noteworthy hypotensive impact.

Associations

Medication: Diuretics (e.g., furosemide, HCTZ, spironolactone), other antihypertensives (e.g., hydralazine, lisinopril, metoprolol, valsartan) may

increment hypotensive impact. NSAIDs (e.g., ibuprofen, naproxen, ketorolac)

may diminish antihypertensive impact. Natural: Herbs with hypotensive

properties (e.g., garlic, ginger, hawthorn) may improve impact. Yohimbe may

decline impact. FOOD: None known. LAB VALUES: May expand serum

BUN, potassium, fatty oils, uric corrosive.

Accessibility (Rx)

Infusion, Emulsion: 50 mL (0.5 mg/mL), 100 mL (0.5 mg/mL), 250-mL vial

(0.5 mg/mL)

Organization/dealing with

IV

Planning

- Do not weaken.

- To guarantee consistency of emulsion, delicately upset vial a few times before use.

- Visually review for particulate matter or staining. Emulsion ought to show up

smooth white. Dispose of if staining or particulate matter is noticed.

Pace of Administration

- Titrate to wanted impact utilizing implantation siphon by means of fringe or focal line.

Capacity

- Refrigerate unused vial in unique container.

- May store at controlled room temperature (77°F) for up to 2 mos.

- Do not freeze.

- Do not get back to fridge once warmed to room temperature. Once the

plug is penetrated, use inside 12 hrs.

- Discard unused parts.

IV incongruencies

Might be controlled with, yet not weakened in, arrangements including Sterile Water

for Injection, 0.9% NaCl, dextrose-containing arrangements, lactated Ringer's, 10%

amino corrosive. Try not to manage with different prescriptions.

Signs/Routes/Dosage

Note: Individualize measurement relying upon wanted B/P and pt reaction. See

producer rules for portion transformation.

Hypertension

IV: ADULTS, ELDERLY: Initiate mixture at 1–2 mg/hr. Titration: Initially, measurement might be multiplied at short (90-sec) spans. As B/P approaches objective, an

expansion in dose ought to be not exactly twofold, and time spans between portion

changes ought to be stretched to q5–10 min. Upkeep: Desired

restorative impact for the most part happens at a pace of 4–6 mg/hr (pts with serious

hypertension might require restricted portions up to 32 mg/hr). Greatest: 16 mg/hr

(close to 21 mg/hr or 1000 mL is prescribed per 24 hrs because of lipid

load).

Dose in Renal Impairment

No portion change.

Dose in Hepatic Impairment

Not indicated; use alert.

Incidental effects

Periodic (6%-3%): Headache, a sleeping disorder, queasiness, retching. Uncommon (not exactly

1%): Syncope, dyspnea.

Antagonistic Effects/Toxic Reactions

May cause atrial fibrillation, hypotension, reflex tachycardia. Bounce back

hypertension might happen in pts who are not changed to oral antihypertensives after cessation. Dihydropyridine calcium channel blockers are known to

have negative inotropic impacts, which might worsen HF. Bounce back

hypertension might cause rising hypertensive emergency, which might cause CVA,

myocardial dead tissue, renal disappointment, HF, seizures.

Nursing Considerations

Benchmark Assessment

Screen for history of flawed lipid digestion, pancreatitis,

hypertriglyceridemia, extreme aortic stenosis; sensitivity to soy items, eggs items. Survey B/P, apical heartbeat preceding commencement.

Mediation/Evaluation

Screen B/P, beat rate. For the most part, an increment of 1–2 mg/hour will create an

extra 2–4 mm Hg decline in systolic B/P. In the event that an oral antihypertensive is

needed to wean off mixture, think about the deferral of beginning of oral drug's

impact. Pts who get delayed IV implantations and are not changed to other

antihypertensives ought to be checked for bounce back hypertension for no less than 8

hrs after end. Acquire serum fatty oil level in pts getting

delayed implantations. Screen for atrial fibrillation, hypotension, reflex

tachycardia; intensification of HF in pts with history of HF. Beta blockers ought to

be ended solely after a progressive decrease in portion.

Patient/Family Teaching

• In certain pts, an oral circulatory strain drug might should be begun;

consistence is vital for control hypertension.

• Life-undermining hypertension emergency might happen up to 8 hrs in the wake of halting

imbuement; report serious uneasiness, chest torment, trouble breathing, migraine, strokelike indications (disarray, trouble talking, loss of motion, uneven shortcoming,

vision misfortune).

clindamycin

klin-da-mye-sin

Apo-Clindamycin

Cleocin

Cleocin T

Cleocin Vaginal

Clindagel

Clindamax

Clindesse

Grouping

PHARMACOTHERAPEUTIC: Lincosamide.

CLINICAL: Antibiotic.

Discovery ALERT

May cause serious, possibly lethal colitis

portrayed by extreme, relentless loose bowels, serious stomach cramps,

section of blood and bodily fluid.

Try not to mistake Cleocin for Clinoril or Cubicin, or clindamycin with clarithromycin, Claritin, or vancomycin.

Employments

Foundational: Treatment of high-impact gram-positive staphylococci and streptococci

(not enterococci), Fusobacterium, Bacteroides spp., and Actinomyces for

treatment of respiratory parcel contaminations, skin/delicate tissue diseases, sepsis, intraabdominal diseases, contaminations of female pelvis and genital plot, bacterial

endocarditis prophylaxis for dental and upper respiratory strategies in

penicillin-hypersensitive pts, perioperative prophylaxis. Skin: Treatment of skin inflammation

vulgaris. Intravaginal: Treatment of bacterial vaginosis. OFF-LABEL:

Treatment of actinomycosis, babesiosis, erysipelas, jungle fever, otitis media,

Pneumocystis jiroveci pneumonia (PCP), sinusitis, toxoplasmosis. PO: Bacterial

vaginosis.

Safety measures

Contraindications: Hypersensitivity to clindamycin. Alerts: Severe hepatic

brokenness; history of GI sickness (particularly colitis).

Activity

Represses protein union of bacterial cell divider by restricting to bacterial ribosomal receptor destinations. Topically, diminishes unsaturated fat focus on skin. Remedial

Impact: Bacteriostatic or bacteriocidal.

Pharmacokinetics

Quickly assimilated from GI plot. Protein restricting: 92%–94%. Broadly disseminated.

Utilized in liver. Basically discharged in pee. Not eliminated by hemodialysis.

Half-life: 1.6–5.3 hrs (expanded in renal/hepatic debilitation, untimely newborn children).

Life expectancy contemplations

Pregnancy/Lactation: Readily crosses placenta. Conveyed in bosom milk.

Effective/vaginal: Unknown whenever conveyed in bosom milk. Youngsters: Caution in

pts more youthful than 1 mo. Old: No age-related safety measures noted.

Connections

Medication: Adsorbent antidiarrheals might defer assimilation. Erythromycin may

increment impact. May expand impacts of neuromuscular blockers (e.g.,

rocuronium, vecuronium). Natural: St. John's wort might diminish

fixation/impact. FOOD: None known. LAB VALUES: May build serum

antacid phosphatase, ALT, AST.

Accessibility (Rx)

Containers: 75 mg, 150 mg, 300 mg. Cream, Vaginal: 2%. Gel,

Effective: 1%. Imbuement, Premix: 300 mg/50 mL, 600 mg/50 mL, 900

mg/50 mL. Infusion Solution: 150 mg/mL. Salve: 1%. Oral

Arrangement: 75 mg/5 mL. Suppositories, Vaginal: 100 mg. Swabs,

Effective: 1%.

Organization/dealing with

IV

Reconstitution

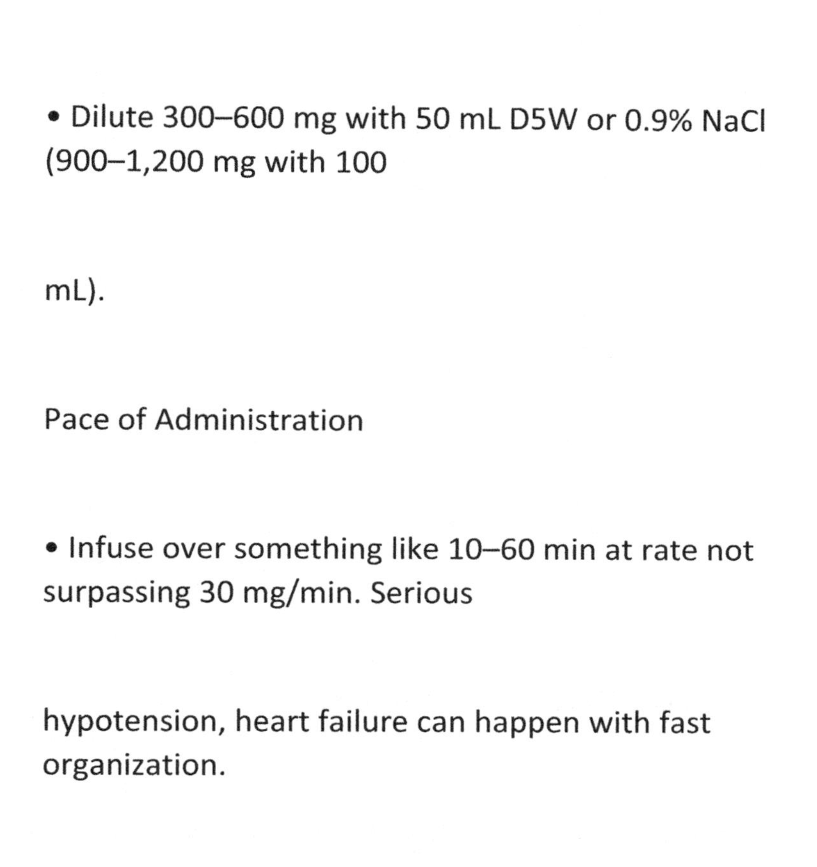

• Dilute 300–600 mg with 50 mL D5W or 0.9% NaCl (900–1,200 mg with 100

mL).

Pace of Administration

• Infuse over something like 10–60 min at rate not surpassing 30 mg/min. Serious

hypotension, heart failure can happen with fast organization.

• No more than 1.2 g ought to be given in a solitary implantation.

Capacity

• Reconstituted IV imbuement (piggyback) is steady for 16 days at room temperature, 32 days whenever refrigerated.

IM

- Do not surpass 600 mg/portion.

- Administer profound IM.

PO

- Store cases at room temperature.

- After reconstitution, oral arrangement is steady for 2 wks at room temperature.

- Do not refrigerate oral arrangement (abstains from thickening).

- Give with no less than 8 oz water (limits esophageal ulceration).

- Give regardless of food.

Effective

- Wash skin; permit to dry totally before application.

- Shake skin cream a long time before each utilization.

- Apply fluid, arrangement, or gel in flimsy film to influenced region.

- Avoid contact with eyes or rubbed regions.

Vaginal, Cream or Suppository

- Use one applicatorful or suppository at sleep time.

- Fill utensil that accompanies cream or suppository to demonstrated level.

- Instruct pt to lie on back with knees drawn vertical and spread separated.

- Insert utensil into vagina and push unclogger to deliver drug.

- Withdraw, wash utensil with cleanser and warm water.

- Wash hands instantly to try not to spread disease.

IV contrary qualities

Allopurinol (Aloprim), fluconazole (Diflucan).

IV Compatibilities

Amiodarone (Cordarone), diltiaZEM (Cardizem), heparin, HYDROmorphone

(Dilaudid), magnesium sulfate, midazolam (Versed), morphine, multivitamins, propofol (Diprivan).

Signs/courses/measurement

Common Dosage

IV, IM: ADULTS, ELDERLY: 600–2,700 mg/day in 2–4 separated dosages.

Most extreme: 4,800 mg/day. Kids 1 MO–16 YRS: 20–40 mg/kg/day in

3–4 separated dosages. Most extreme: 2,700 mg/day. Kids YOUNGER

THAN 1 MO: 5 mg/kg/portion q6–12h.

PO: ADULTS, ELDERLY: 150–450 mg q6h. Most extreme: 1,800 mg/day.

Kids 1 MO–16 YRS: (Capsule): 8–40 mg/kg/day in separated portions q6–

8h. Most extreme: 1,800 mg/day. (Oral Solution): 8–25 mg/kg/day in 3–4 separated

dosages. Least portion: 37.5 mg multiple times/day. Kids YOUNGER THAN

1 MO: 5 mg/kg/portion q6–12h.

Bacterial Vaginosis

Intravaginal (Cream): ADULTS: One applicatorful at sleep time for 3–7 days or

1 suppository at sleep time for 3 days. (Clindesse): ADULTS: One applicatorful

when every day.

Skin inflammation Vulgaris

Effective: ADULTS: Apply slender layer to influenced region twice day by day.

Dose in Renal/Hepatic Impairment

No portion change.

Incidental effects

Incessant: Systemic: Abdominal torment, queasiness, spewing, looseness of the bowels. Effective: Dry,

textured skin. Vaginal: Vaginitis, pruritus. Intermittent: Systemic: Phlebitis; torment,

induration at IM infusion site; unfavorably susceptible response, urticaria, pruritus. Effective:

Contact dermatitis, stomach torment, gentle the runs, consuming, stinging. Vaginal:

Migraine, wooziness, sickness, retching, stomach torment. Uncommon: Vaginal:

Extreme touchiness response.

Unfavorable impacts/harmful responses

Anti-infection related colitis, different superinfections (stomach cramps, serious

watery loose bowels, fever) may happen during and a few wks after clindamycin

treatment (counting skin structure). Blood dyscrasias (leukopenia,

thrombocytopenia), nephrotoxicity (proteinuria, azotemia, oliguria) happen seldom.

Thrombophlebitis with IV organization.

Nursing contemplations

Benchmark evaluation

Get pattern WBC. Question pt for history of hypersensitivities. Keep away from, if conceivable,

simultaneous utilization of neuromuscular hindering specialists.

Mediation/assessment

Screen every day example of gut movement, stool consistency. Report looseness of the bowels

expeditiously because of potential for genuine colitis (even with effective or vaginal

organization). Evaluate skin for rash (dryness, disturbance) with effective application.

With all courses of organization, be ready for superinfection: fever, spewing, the runs, butt-centric/genital pruritus, oral mucosal changes (ulceration, torment,

erythema).

Patient/family educating

- Continue treatment for full length of treatment.

- Doses ought to be equitably dispersed.

- Take oral portions with something like 8 oz water.

- Use alert while applying effective clindamycin simultaneously with stripping or

rough skin inflammation specialists, cleansers, liquor containing beauty care products to stay away from total impact.

- Do not make a difference effective arrangements close to eyes, scraped regions.

- Report serious industrious looseness of the bowels, cramps, bleeding stool.

- Vaginal: In occasion of unplanned contact with eyes, wash with a lot of

cool faucet water.

- Do not take part in sex during treatment.

- Wear sterile cushion to ensure garments against stains. Tampons ought not be

utilized.

cloBAZam

kloe-ba-zam

Apo-CloBAZam

Novo-CloBAZam

Onfi

Arrangement

PHARMACOTHERAPEUTIC: Benzodiazepine (Schedule IV).

CLINICAL: Anticonvulsant.

Try not to mistake cloBAZam for clonazePAM or cloZAPine.

Employments

Adjunctive treatment of seizures related with Lennox-Gastaut condition in

pts 2 yrs old enough and more seasoned. OFF-LABEL: Catamenial epilepsy; epilepsy

(monotherapy).

Safeguards

Contraindications: Hypersensitivity to cloBAZam. Alerts: Elderly,

incapacitated, gentle to direct hepatic impedance, previous muscle shortcoming

or then again ataxia, attending CNS depressants, weakened gag reflex, respiratory

sickness, rest apnea, associative poor CYP2C19 metabolizers, pts in danger for falls, myasthenia gravis, thin point glaucoma.

Activity

Potentiates neurotransmission of gamma-aminobutyric corrosive (GABA) by restricting

to GABA receptor. Pushes down nerve drive transmission in engine cortex.

Restorative Effect: Decreases seizure movement.

Pharmacokinetics

Quickly consumed after PO organization. Used in liver. Pinnacle plasma

focus: 0.5–4 hrs. Protein restricting: 80–90%. Fundamentally discharged in pee.

Obscure whenever eliminated by dialysis. Half-life: 36–42 hrs.

Life expectancy contemplations

Pregnancy/Lactation: Excreted in bosom milk. Hormonal contraceptives may

have diminished adequacy. Nonhormonal contraception suggested.

Kids: Safety and adequacy not set up in pts more youthful than 2 yrs. Older:

May have diminished freedom levels (starting portion 5 mg/day).

Communications

Medication: CYP2C19 inhibitors (e.g., fluconazole, fluvoxaMINE, omeprazole,

ticlopidine) may expand focus/impacts. Liquor, other CNS

depressants (e.g., lorazepam, morphine, zolpidem) may expand CNS

sorrow. May diminish impacts of hormonal contraceptives.

Natural: Gotu kola, kava, St. John's wort, valerian might increment

CNS wretchedness. St. John's wort might diminish impacts. FOOD: None known.

LAB VALUES: None huge.

clomiPRAMINE

kloe-mip-rah-meen

Anafranil

Apo-ClomiPRAMINE

Novo-ClomiPRAMINE

Grouping

PHARMACOTHERAPEUTIC: Tricyclic.

CLINICAL: Antidepressant.

■ BLACK BOX ALERT ■ Increased danger of self-destructive ideation and conduct

in youngsters, teenagers, youthful grown-ups 18–24 yrs with significant burdensome

jumble, other mental problems.

Try not to mistake Anafranil for enalapril, or clomiPRAMINE with chlorproMAZINE, clevidipine, clomiPHENE, or desipramine.

Employments

Treatment of over the top habitual problem. OFF-LABEL: Depression, alarm

assaults.

Precautionary measures

Contraindications: Hypersensitivity to clomiPRAMINE, other tricyclic specialists.

Intense recuperation period after MI, utilization of MAOIs expected for mental problems

(simultaneously or inside 14 days of suspending either clomipramine or MAOI).

Commencement in pts getting linezolid or methylene blue. Alerts: Pts at high danger

for self destruction, prostatic hypertrophy, history of urinary maintenance/deterrent,

limited point glaucoma, seizures, cardiovascular/hepatic/renal illness,

hyperthyroidism, liquor addiction, xerostomia, visual issues, old, obstruction,

history of inside impediment. Cancers of the adrenal medulla (e.g.,

pheochromocytoma).

Activity

Squares reuptake of synapses (norepinephrine, serotonin) at CNS presynaptic layers, expanding accessibility at postsynaptic receptor locales.

Restorative Effect: Reduces over the top habitual conduct.

Pharmacokinetics

Quickly assimilated. Used in liver. Wiped out in pee (51%–60%), excrement

(24%–32%). Half-life: 20–30 hrs.

Life expectancy contemplations

Pregnancy/Lactation: Distributed in bosom milk. Kids: Increased danger of

self-destructive ideation, conduct noted in kids, young people. Wellbeing and adequacy in pts more youthful than 10 yrs not set up. Older: Not

prescribed in older because of anticholinergic impacts, potential for sedation,

orthostatic hypotension.

Associations

Medication: Alcohol, other CNS depressants (e.g., lorazepam, morphine,

zolpidem) may build CNS, respiratory melancholy, hypotensive impact.

Cimetidine, haloperidol might expand focus, hazard of harmfulness. May

decline impacts of cloNIDine. PHENobarbital might diminish focus, stimulant impact. MAOIs (e.g., phenelzine, selegiline) may build hazard of

neuroleptic dangerous disorder, seizures, hyperpyresis, hypertensive emergency.

Phenothiazines (e.g., chlorpromazine, thioridazine) may increment

anticholinergic, narcotic impacts. Sympathomimetics (e.g., dopamine,

norepinephrine) may expand the danger of heart impacts. Natural: Gota kola,

kava, SAMe, St. John's wort, valerian might expand CNS sorrow.

FOOD: Grapefruit items might build focus, poisonousness. LAB

Qualities: May modify serum glucose, ECG readings.

Accessibility (Rx)

Containers: 25 mg, 50 mg, 75 mg.

Organization/dealing with

PO

• May give with food to diminish hazard of GI unsettling influence.

• Recommend sleep time organization.

Signs/courses/measurements

NOTE: Following portion titration, may give once-day by day portion at sleep time.

Over the top Compulsive Disorder (OCD)

PO: ADULTS, ELDERLY: Initially, 25 mg/day. May steadily increment to 100

mg/day in separated dosages in the initial 2 wks. Most extreme: 250 mg/day.

Kids 10 YRS AND OLDER: Initially, 25 mg/day. May progressively

increment up to limit of 3 mg/kg/day or 100 mg in separated dosages (whichever

is least). Upkeep: May additionally increment to 3 mg/kg or 200 mg/day

(whichever is less).

Dose in Renal/Hepatic Impairment

Use alert.

Incidental effects

Incessant (30%–15%): Ejaculatory disappointment, dry mouth, drowsiness, quakes,

dazedness, cerebral pain, obstruction, exhaustion, sickness. Incidental (14%–5%):

Barrenness, diaphoresis, dyspepsia, sexual brokenness, dysmenorrhea,

anxiety, weight acquire, pharyngitis. Uncommon (under 5%): Diarrhea, myalgia,

rhinitis, expanded hunger, paresthesia, memory weakness, tension, rash,

pruritus, anorexia, stomach torment, regurgitating, fart, flushing, UTI, back

torment.

Unfriendly impacts/poisonous responses

Excess might create seizures, cardiovascular impacts (extreme orthostatic

hypotension, tipsiness, tachycardia, palpitations, arrhythmias), changed

temperature guideline (hyperpyrexia, hypothermia). Unexpected cessation

after delayed treatment might deliver cerebral pain, disquietude, queasiness, regurgitating, clear

dreams. Paleness, agranulocytosis have been noted.

Nursing contemplations

Benchmark evaluation

Survey mental status, thought content, level of interest, mind-set, conduct, self-destructive ideation.

Intercession/assessment

Administer self-destructive danger pt intently during early treatment (as sadness diminishes,

energy level improves, expanding self destruction potential). Survey appearance,

conduct, discourse design, level of interest, state of mind.

Patient/family instructing

• May cause dry mouth, clogging, obscured vision. Stay away from undertakings that require

readiness, engine abilities until reaction to medicate is set up.

• Tolerance to postural hypotension, soothing, anticholinergic impacts ordinarily

create during early treatment.

• Maximum restorative impact might be noted in 2–4 wks.

• Do not suddenly suspend drug.

• Daily portion might be given at sleep time to limit daytime sedation.

• Avoid liquor.

• Report deteriorating sorrow, self-destructive ideation, change in conduct.

clonazePAM

kloe-naz-e-pam

Apo-ClonazePAM

KlonoPIN

Rivotril

Characterization

PHARMACOTHERAPEUTIC: Benzodiazepine (Schedule IV).

CLINICAL: Anticonvulsant, antianxiety.

■ BLACK BOX ALERT ■ Concomitant use with narcotics might result in

significant sedation, respiratory wretchedness, trance state, and passing.

Try not to befuddle clonazePAM or KlonoPIN with cloBAZam, cloNIDine,

cloZAPine, or LORazepam.

Employments

Assistant in treatment of Lennox-Gastaut condition (petit mal variation epilepsy);

akinetic, myoclonic seizures; nonappearance seizures (petit mal) inert to

succinimides. Treatment of frenzy problem. OFF-LABEL: Burning mouth

condition, REM rest conduct issue, fundamental quake.

Safeguards

Contraindications: Hypersensitivity to clonazePAM. Dynamic tight point

glaucoma, serious hepatic infection, pregnancy. Alerts: Renal/hepatic

hindrance, weakened gag reflex, constant respiratory infection, older, incapacitated

pts, melancholy, pts in danger of self destruction or medication reliance, attendant utilization of

other CNS depressants.

Activity

Pushes down all degrees of CNS; pushes down nerve drive transmission in engine

cortex. Stifles strange release in petit mal seizures. Restorative

Impact: Produces anxiolytic, anticonvulsant impacts.

Pharmacokinetics

Course Onset Peak Duration

PO 20–60 min — 12 hrs or less

All around retained from GI lot. Protein restricting: 85%. Used in liver.

Discharged in pee. Not eliminated by hemodialysis. Half-life: 18–50 hrs.

Life expectancy contemplations

Pregnancy/Lactation: Crosses placenta. Might be appropriated in bosom milk.

Constant ingestion during pregnancy might deliver withdrawal side effects, CNS sadness in youngsters. Kids: Long-term use may unfavorably influence

physical/mental turn of events. Older: Not prescribed in old due to

anticholinergic impacts, potential for sedation, orthostatic hypotension.

Communications

Medication: Alcohol, other CNS depressants (e.g., lorazepam, morphine,

zolpidem) may build CNS depressant impact. CYP3A4 inhibitors (e.g., azole

antifungals) may build focus, harmfulness. Home grown: Gotu kola, kava

kava, SAMe, St. John's wort, valerian might build CNS sorrow. St.

John's wort might diminish fixation/impacts. FOOD: None known. LAB

Qualities: None huge.

Accessibility (Rx)

Tablets (Klonopin): 0.5 mg, 1 mg, 2 mg. Tablets (Orally Disintegrating):

0.125 mg, 0.25 mg, 0.5 mg, 1 mg, 2 mg.

Organization/taking care of

PO

- Give regardless of food.

- Swallow entire with water.

Orally Disintegrating Tablet

- Open pocket, strip back foil; don't push tablet through foil.

- Remove tablet with dry hands, place in mouth.

- Swallow with or without water.

- Use following eliminating from bundle.

Signs/courses/measurements

Seizures

PO: ADULTS, ELDERLY, CHILDREN 10 YRS AND OLDER: Initial portion not to surpass 1.5 mg/day in 3 isolated dosages; might be expanded in 0.5-to 1-mg

augments at regular intervals until seizures are controlled or antagonistic impacts happen.

Support: 2–8 mg/day in 1–2 separated dosages. Greatest: 20 mg/day.

Babies, CHILDREN YOUNGER THAN 10 YRS OR WEIGHING LESS

THAN 30 KG: 0.01–0.03 mg/kg/day (greatest starting portion: 0.05 mg/kg/day)

in 2–3 separated portions; might be expanded by close to 0.25–0.5 mg each 3

days until seizures are controlled or antagonistic impacts happen. Upkeep: 0.1–0.2

mg/kg/day in 3 separated dosages. Most extreme: 0.2 mg/kg/day.

Frenzy Disorder

PO: ADULTS, ELDERLY: Initially, 0.25 mg twice every day. Expansion in

additions of 0.125–0.25 mg twice day by day at regular intervals. Target portion: 1 mg/day.

Most extreme: 4 mg/day. Note: Discontinue progressively by 0.125 mg twice every day

q3days until totally removed.

Measurement in Renal Impairment

Use alert.

Dose in Hepatic Impairment

Gentle to direct weakness: Use with alert. Extreme weakness:

Contraindicated.

Incidental effects

Successive (37%–11%): Mild, transient sleepiness; ataxia, conduct

unsettling influences (hostility, touchiness, fomentation), esp. in youngsters. Intermittent

(10%–5%): Dizziness, ataxia, URI, weakness. Uncommon (4% or less): Impaired

memory, dysarthria, apprehension, sinusitis, rhinitis, clogging, unfavorably susceptible

response.

Unfavorable impacts/poisonous responses

Unexpected withdrawal might bring about articulated fretfulness, touchiness, sleep deprivation,

hand quakes, stomach/muscle cramps, diaphoresis, retching, status

epilepticus. Excess outcomes in laziness, disarray, reduced reflexes,

extreme lethargies. Remedy: Flumazenil (see Appendix J for measurements).

Nursing contemplations

Pattern evaluation

Audit history of seizure issue (recurrence, term, power, level of

awareness [LOC]). For fit of anxiety, survey engine reactions (tumult, shuddering, pressure), autonomic reactions (cold/damp hands, diaphoresis).

Intercession/assessment

Notice for abundance sedation, respiratory discouragement, self-destructive ideation. Evaluate

youngsters, older for confusing response, especially during early treatment.

Start seizure safeguards, notice often for repeat of seizure action.

Help with ambulation if sluggishness, ataxia happen. For pts on long haul treatment,

CBC, BMP, LFT ought to be performed occasionally. Assess for helpful reaction: diminished force and recurrence of seizures or then again, whenever utilized in alarm

assault, quiet look, diminished anxiety.

Patient/family educating

• Avoid undertakings that require readiness, engine abilities until reaction to sedate is

set up.

• Do not unexpectedly end medicine after long haul treatment.

• Strict support of medication treatment is fundamental for seizure control.

• Avoid liquor.

• Report gloom, considerations of self destruction/self-hurt, extreme laziness, GI indications, declining or loss of seizure control.

cloNIDine

klon-I-deen

Apo-CloNIDine

Catapres

Catapres-TTS

Dixarit

Duraclon

Kapvay

Novo-CloNIDine

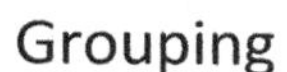

Grouping

PHARMACOTHERAPEUTIC: Alpha2

- adrenergic agonist.

CLINICAL: Antihypertensive.

■ BLACK BOX ALERT ■ Epidural: Not to be utilized for perioperative,

obstetric, or post pregnancy torment. Should weaken concentrated epidural injectable

(500 mcg/mL) preceding use.

Try not to mistake Catapres for Cataflam, or cloNIDine with clomiPHENE,

clonazepam, KlonoPIN, or quiNIDine.

Employments

Quick Release, Transdermal Patch: Treatment of hypertension alone or

in blend with other antihypertensive specialists. Kapvay: Treatment of

consideration deficiency hyperactivity issue (ADHD). Epidural: Combined with

narcotics for help of extreme malignancy torment. OFF-LABEL: Opioid or nicotine

withdrawal, counteraction of headache migraines, treatment of loose bowels in diabetes

mellitus, treatment of dysmenorrhea, menopausal flushing, liquor reliance, glaucoma, cloZAPine-incited sialorrhea, Tourette's disorder, sleep deprivation in

youngsters.

Safeguards

Contraindications: Hypersensitivity to cloNIDine. Epidural: Contraindicated

in pts with draining diathesis or disease at the infusion site; pts getting

anticoagulation treatment. Alerts: Depression, old. Serious coronary

deficiency, late MI, cerebrovascular sickness, persistent renal weakness,

previous bradycardia, sinus hub brokenness, conduction aggravations;

simultaneous use with digoxin, diltiaZEM, metoprolol, verapamil.

Activity

Animates alpha2

- adrenergic receptors, lessening thoughtful CNS reaction.

Epidural: Prevents torment signal transmission to cerebrum and produces absense of pain at

pre-and post-alpha-adrenergic receptors in spinal rope. ADHD: Mechanism of

activity obscure. Helpful Effect: Reduces fringe opposition; diminishes

B/P, pulse. Produces absense of pain.

Pharmacokinetics

Course Onset Peak Duration

PO 0.5–1 hr 2–4 hrs 6–10 hrs

Very much consumed from GI parcel. Transdermal best ingested from chest and upper

arm; least ingested from thigh. Protein restricting: 20%–40%. Utilized in liver.

Principally discharged in pee. Negligibly eliminated by hemodialysis. Half-life: 6–

20 hrs (expanded in renal weakness).

Life expectancy contemplations

Pregnancy/Lactation: Crosses placenta. Conveyed in bosom milk. Youngsters:

More delicate to impacts; use alert. Old: Not suggested in older due

to high danger of CNS unfriendly impacts, orthostatic hypotension. Stay away from as first-line

antihypertensive.

Cooperations

Medication: Discontinuation of simultaneous beta-blocker (e.g., carvedilol,

metoprolol) treatment might build hazard of cloNIDine-withdrawal hypertensive

emergency. Tricyclic antidepressants (e.g., amitriptyline, doxepin, nortriptyline)

may diminish impact (may require expanded portion of cloNIDine). Digoxin, diltiaZEM, metoprolol, verapamil might expand hazard of genuine bradycardia.

Home grown: Gotu kola, kava, SAMe, St. John's wort, valerian may

increment CNS despondency. Ephedra, ginseng, yohimbe may diminish

antihypertensive impact. FOOD: None known. LAB VALUES: None critical.

Accessibility (Rx)

Infusion Solution (Duraclon): 100 mcg/mL, 500 mcg/mL. Tablets

(Catapres): 0.1 mg, 0.2 mg, 0.3 mg. (Kapvay): 0.1 mg, 0.2 mg. Transdermal

Fix (Catapres-TTS): 2.5 mg (discharge at 0.1 mg/24 hrs), 5 mg (discharge at 0.2

mg/24 hrs), 7.5 mg (discharge at 0.3 mg/24 hrs).

Broadened Release Tablets:(Kapvay): 0.1 mg.

Organization/dealing with

PO

- Give regardless of food.

- Tablets might be squashed.

- Give last oral portion not long before sleep time.

- Swallow broadened discharge tablets entire; don't break, pulverize, disintegrate, or

partition.

Transdermal

• Apply transdermal framework to dry, bare space of flawless skin on upper arm or

chest.

• Rotate locales (forestalls skin disturbance).

• Do not manage fix to change portion.

Epidural

• Must be regulated simply by clinical work force prepared in epidural

the board.

IV inconsistencies

None known.

IV Compatibilities

Bupivacaine (Marcaine, Sensorcaine), fentaNYL (Sublimaze), heparin, ketamine

(Ketalar), lidocaine, LORazepam (Ativan).

Signs/courses/measurement

Hypertension

PO: ADULTS: (Immediate Release): Initially, 0.1 mg two times every day. Increment by

0.1–0.2 mg q2–4days. Upkeep: 0.2–1.2 mg/day in 2–4 split portions to

limit of 2.4 mg/day. Old: Initially, 0.1 mg at sleep time. May increment bit by bit. Youngsters 12 YRS AND OLDER: Initially, 0.2 mg/day in 2

isolated dosages. May increment bit by bit at 5-to 7-day stretches in 0.1 mg/day

increases. Greatest: 2.4 mg/day.

Transdermal: ADULTS, ELDERLY: Initially, framework conveying 0.1 mg/24 hrs

applied once q7days. May increment by 0.1 mg at 1-to 2-wk spans. Regular

dose range: 0.1–0.3 mg once wkly.

Intense Hypertension

PO: ADULTS: Initially, 0.1–0.2 mg followed by 0.1 mg each hr if essential,

up to most extreme absolute portion of 0.7 mg.

Consideration Deficit Hyperactivity Disorder (ADHD)

PO: CHILDREN 45 KG OR LESS: (Immediate Release): Initially 0.05

mg/day at sleep time. May increment in augmentations of 0.05 mg/day q3–7days up to

0.2 mg/day (27–40.5 kg), 0.3 mg/day (40.5–45 kg). More noteworthy THAN 45 KG:

(Prompt Release): 0.1 mg at sleep time. May increment 0.1 mg/day q3–7 days.

Most extreme: 0.4 mg/day. Expanded Release Tablet (Kapvay): CHILDREN 6

YRS AND OLDER: Initially, 0.1 mg every day at sleep time. May increment in additions of 0.1 mg/day at wkly stretches (Maximum: 0.4 mg/day). Dosages

ought to be taken twice every day with higher split portion given at sleep time.

Extreme Pain

Epidural: ADULTS, ELDERLY: 30–40 mcg/hr. Kids: Range: 0.5–2

mcg/kg/hr, not to surpass grown-up portion.

Measurement in Renal/Hepatic Impairment

No portion change.

Incidental effects

Continuous (40%–10%): Dry mouth, languor, tipsiness, sedation, obstruction. Infrequent (5%–1%): Tablets, Injection: Depression, pedal

edema, loss of craving, diminished sexual capacity, tingling eyes, tipsiness,

queasiness, spewing, apprehension. Transdermal: Pruritus, redness or obscuring of

skin. Uncommon (under 1%): Nightmares, distinctive dreams, sensation of chilliness in

distal limits (esp. the digits).

Unfriendly impacts/poisonous responses

Excess produces significant hypotension, touchiness, bradycardia, respiratory

sadness, hypothermia, miosis (pupillary tightening), arrhythmias, apnea.

Sudden withdrawal might bring about bounce back hypertension related with

apprehension, fomentation, nervousness, sleep deprivation, paresthesia, quake, flushing,

diaphoresis. May deliver sedation in pts with intense CVA.

Nursing contemplations

Pattern evaluation

Acquire B/P preceding each portion is managed, notwithstanding customary

observing (be aware of B/P vacillations).

Intercession/assessment

Screen B/P, beat, mental status. Screen day by day example of gut movement, stool

consistency. In case cloNIDine is to be removed, suspend simultaneous betablocker treatment a few days prior to ending cloNIDine (forestalls

cloNIDine withdrawal hypertensive emergency). Gradually decrease cloNIDine dose

more than 2–4 days.

Patient/family instructing

• Sugarless gum, tastes of water might ease dry mouth.

• Avoid assignments that require sharpness, engine abilities until reaction to tranquilize is

set up.

- To decrease hypotensive impact, rise gradually from misleading standing.

- Skipping portions or intentionally ending medication might deliver extreme bounce back

hypertension.

- Avoid liquor.

- If fix slackens during 7-day application period, secure with cement cover.

clopidogrel

kloe-pid-gracious grel

Apo-Clopidogrel

Plavix

Order

PHARMACOTHERAPEUTIC: Thienopyridine subordinate.

CLINICAL: Antiplatelet.

■ BLACK BOX ALERT ■ Diminished adequacy in CYP2C19

metabolizers expands hazard for cardiovascular occasions. Pts with CYP2C19*2

as well as CYP2C19*3 alleles might have diminished platelet hindrance.

Try not to mistake Plavix for Elavil or Paxil.

Employments

To diminish pace of MI and stroke in pts with non–ST-section rise intense coronary condition (ACS), intense ST-rise MI (STEMI); pts with history of

late MI or stroke, set up fringe blood vessel infection (PAD). OFFLABEL: Graft patency (saphenous vein), stable coronary course infection (in

mix with headache medicine). Starting treatment of ACS in pts susceptible to ibuprofen.

Insurances

Contraindications: Hypersensitivity to clopidogrel. Dynamic dying (e.g.,

peptic ulcer, intracranial discharge). Alerts: Severe hepatic/renal

disability, pts in danger of expanded dying (e.g., injury), simultaneous utilization of anticoagulants. Keep away from simultaneous utilization of CYP2C19 inhibitors (e.g., omeprazole).

Activity

Hinders restricting of chemical adenosine phosphate (ADP) to its platelet receptor

also, ensuing ADP-interceded enactment of a glycoprotein complex.

Helpful Effect: Inhibits platelet accumulation.

Pharmacokinetics

Course Onset Peak Duration

PO 2 hrs 5–7 days (with rehashed portions of 75 mg/day) 5 days after last portion

Quickly retained. Protein restricting: 98%. Processed in liver. Disposed of similarly in the pee and excrement. Half-life: 8 hrs.

Life expectancy contemplations

Pregnancy/Lactation: Unknown if drug crosses placenta or is dispersed in

bosom milk. Kids: Safety and adequacy not set up. Older: No agerelated safety measures noted.

Connections

Medication: Aspirin, NSAIDs (e.g., ibuprofen, ketorolac, naproxen), warfarin

may expand hazard of dying. Proton siphon inhibitors (e.g., omeprazole,

pantoprazole) may diminish viability, increment hazard of cardiovascular occasions.

Home grown: Cat's hook, dong quai, evening primrose, feverfew, garlic, ginger,

ginkgo, ginseng, green tea, red clover might have added substance antiplatelet impacts.

FOOD: Grapefruit items might diminish impacts. LAB VALUES: May

increment serum bilirubin, ALT, AST, cholesterol, uric corrosive. May diminish

neutrophil count, platelet count.

Accessibility (Rx)

Tablets: 75 mg, 300 mg.

Organization/dealing with

PO

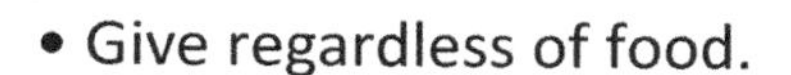

• Give regardless of food.

• Avoid grapefruit items.

Signs/courses/measurements

Ongoing MI, Stroke, PAD

PO: ADULTS, ELDERLY: 75 mg once day by day.

Intense Coronary Syndrome (ACS), Unstable Angina/NSTEMI

PO: ADULTS, ELDERLY: Initially, stacking portion of 300–600 mg, then, at that point 75 mg

when day by day (in mix with headache medicine for as long as a year, then, at that point ibuprofen

endlessly).

ACS (STEMI)

Note: Continue for something like 14 days as long as a year.

PO: ADULTS, ELDERLY 75 YRS OR YOUNGER: Initially 300-mg stacking

portion, then, at that point 75 mg once every day. Old OLDER THAN 75 YRS: 75 mg once

every day.

ACS (PCI)

PO: ADULTS, ELDERLY: Initially, 600 mg, then, at that point 75 mg once every day (in

mix with anti-inflamatory medicine) for somewhere around a year.

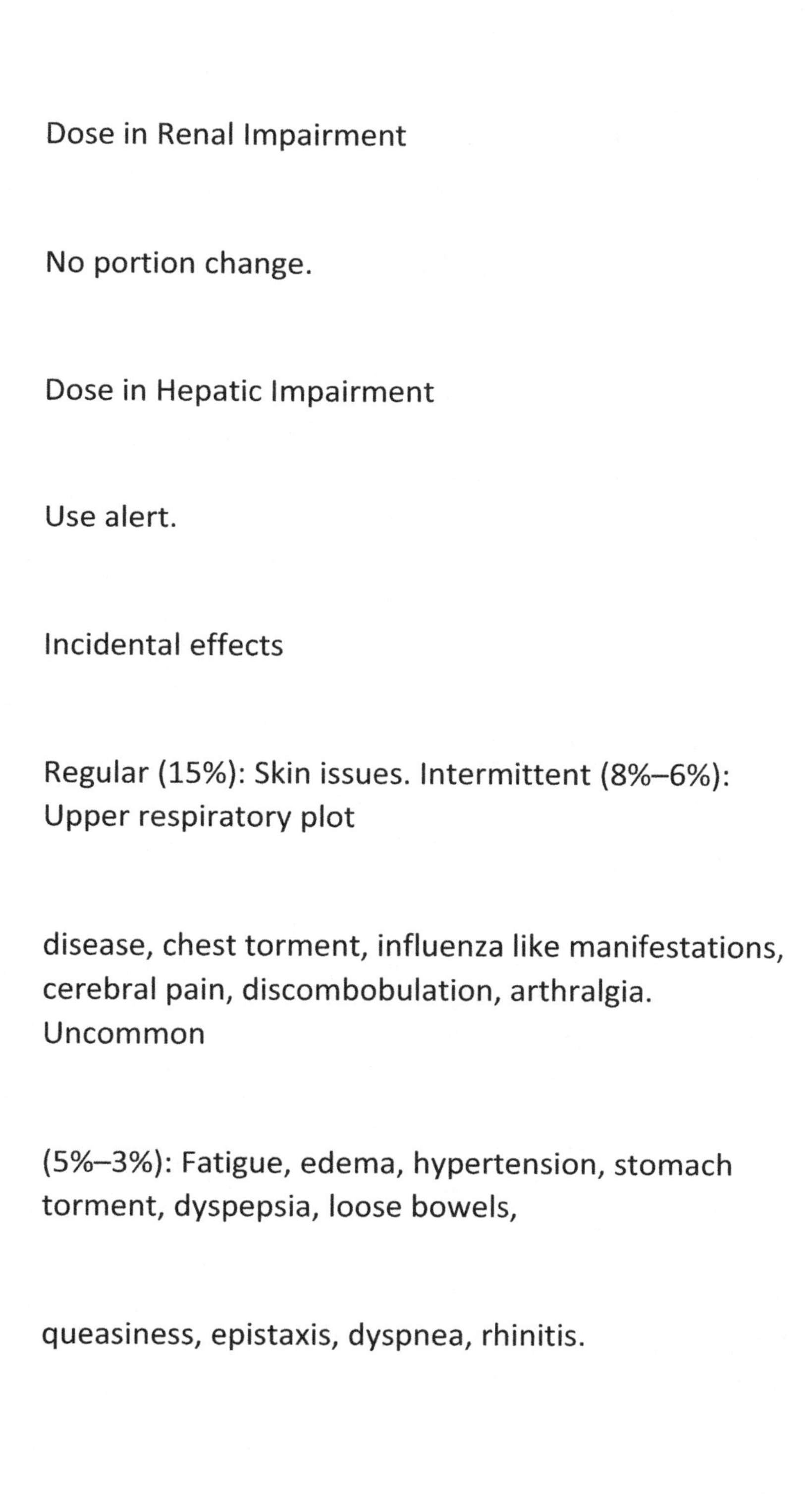

Dose in Renal Impairment

No portion change.

Dose in Hepatic Impairment

Use alert.

Incidental effects

Regular (15%): Skin issues. Intermittent (8%–6%): Upper respiratory plot

disease, chest torment, influenza like manifestations, cerebral pain, discombobulation, arthralgia. Uncommon

(5%–3%): Fatigue, edema, hypertension, stomach torment, dyspepsia, loose bowels,

queasiness, epistaxis, dyspnea, rhinitis.

Unfavorable impacts/harmful responses

Agranulocytosis, aplastic frailty/pancytopenia, thrombotic thrombocytopenic

purpura (TTP) happen once in a while. Hepatitis, touchiness response, anaphylactoid

response have been accounted for.

Nursing contemplations

Gauge evaluation

Acquire pattern sciences, platelet count, PFA. Perform platelet counts previously

drug treatment, q2days during first wk of treatment, and wkly from there on until

helpful support portion is reached. Unexpected end of medication treatment produces raised platelet count inside 5 days.

Intercession/assessment

Screen platelet count for proof of thrombocytopenia. Evaluate Hgb, Hct, for

proof of dying; serum ALT, AST, bilirubin, BUN, creatinine;

signs/manifestations of hepatic deficiency during treatment.

Patient/family educating

- It might require some investment to quit draining during drug treatment.

- Report any surprising dying.

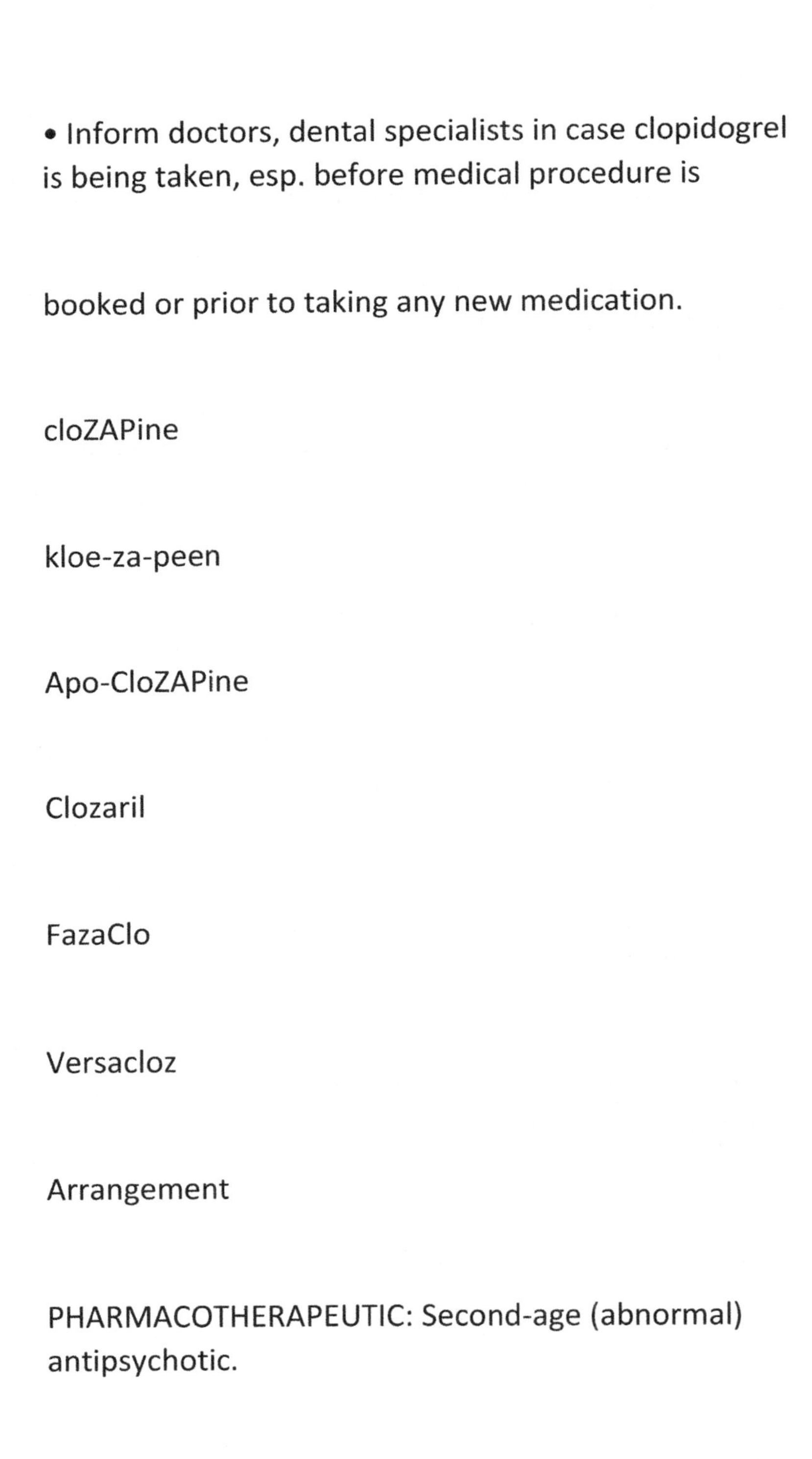

• Inform doctors, dental specialists in case clopidogrel is being taken, esp. before medical procedure is

booked or prior to taking any new medication.

cloZAPine

kloe-za-peen

Apo-CloZAPine

Clozaril

FazaClo

Versacloz

Arrangement

PHARMACOTHERAPEUTIC: Second-age (abnormal) antipsychotic.

CLINICAL: Antipsychotic.

■ BLACK BOX ALERT ■ Significant danger of perilous

agranulocytosis, expanded danger of possibly lethal cardiovascular occasions,

especially myocarditis, in older pts with dementia-related psychosis.

May cause extreme orthostatic hypotension, bradycardia, syncope, cardiovascular

capture, portion subordinate seizures.

Try not to mistake cloZAPine for clonazePAM, cloNIDine, or KlonoPIN, or

Clozaril with Clinoril or Colazal.

Employments

The board of seriously sick schizophrenic pts who have neglected to react to

other antipsychotic treatment. Treatment of repetitive self-destructive conduct in

schizophrenia or schizoaffective problem. OFF-LABEL: Schizoaffective

jumble, bipolar confusion, youth psychosis, fanatical habitual issue,

unsettling identified with Alzheimer's dementia.

Safety measures

Contraindications: Hypersensitivity to cloZAPine. History of cloZAPineinduced agranulocytosis or extreme granulocytopenia. Alerts: History of seizures, cardiovascular sickness, myocarditis, respiratory/hepatic/renal

impedance, liquor withdrawal, high danger of self destruction, crippled ileus, myasthenia

gravis, pts in danger for goal pneumonia, urinary maintenance, thin point

glaucoma, prostatic hypertrophy, xerostomia, visual unsettling influences, blockage,

history of gut hindrance, diabetes mellitus. History of long QT

prolongation/ventricular arrhythmias; attending utilization of meds that

draw out QT span; hypokalemia, hypomagnesemia.

Activity

Meddles with restricting of DOPamine and serotonin receptor destinations. Remedial

Impact: Diminishes schizophrenic conduct.

Pharmacokinetics

Promptly assimilated from GI plot. Protein restricting: 97%. Utilized in liver.

Discharged in pee. Half-life: 12 hrs.

Life expectancy contemplations

Pregnancy/Lactation: Crosses placenta. Avoid use during pregnancy.

Dispersed in bosom milk. Breastfeeding not suggested. Youngsters: Not

suggested for use. Older: Avoid use in pts with dementia.

Connections

Medication: Antihypertensive prescriptions (e.g., amLODIPine, lisinopril,

valsartan) may build hazard of hypotension. Liquor, other CNS

depressants (e.g., lorazepam, morphine, zolpidem) may build CNS

depressant impacts. Bone marrow depressants might build myelosuppression.

Cimetidine, citalopram, ciprofloxacin, erythromycin might increment

focus, hazard of antagonistic impacts. SSRIs (e.g., PARoxetine) may increment focus. Lithium might expand hazard of disarray, dyskinesia, seizures.

Drugs drawing out QT stretch (e.g., amiodarone, azithromycin,

ciprofloxacin, haloperidol) may expand hazard of QT prolongation. CYP3A4

inducers (e.g., phenytoin, carBAMazepine, rifAMPin) may diminish

fixation/impacts. Home grown: St. John's wort might diminish

focus/helpful impacts. Kava, gotu kola, valerian, St. John's

wort might expand hazard of CNS misery. FOOD: None known. LAB

Qualities: May build serum glucose, cholesterol (uncommon), fatty substances (uncommon).

Accessibility (Rx)

Suspension, Oral (Versacloz): 50 mg/mL (100 mL). Tablets (Clozaril): 25 mg,

50 mg, 100 mg, 200 mg. Tablets (Orally Disintegrating [FazaClo]): 12.5 mg,

25 mg, 100 mg, 150 mg, 200 mg.

Organization/dealing with

PO

• Give regardless of food.

• Suspension: Use oral needles (gave). Shake well, regulate portion following planning. Suspension stable for 100 days after beginning jug

opening.

Orally Disintegrating Tablets

- Remove from foil rankle; don't push tablet through foil.

- Remove tablet with dry hands, place in mouth.

- Allow to disintegrate in mouth; swallow with spit.

- If portion requires parting tablet, dispose of unused piece.